The Fastest Keto Diet Breakfast Cookbook

Delicious Recipes affordable for

Busy People and Beginners

Otis Fisher

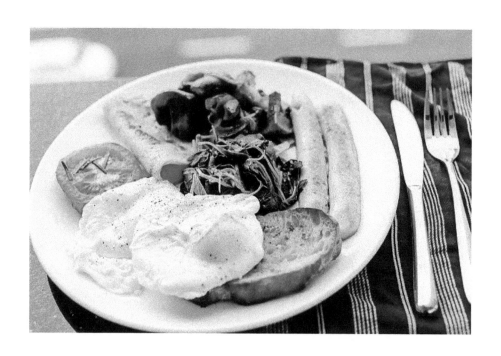

advice. The content within this book has been derived from various sources. Please consult a licensed professional before attempting any techniques outlined in this book.

By reading this document, the reader agrees that under no circumstances is the author responsible for any losses, direct or indirect, which are incurred as a result of the use of information contained within this document, including, but not limited to, — errors, omissions, or inaccuracies.

Tables of content

Breakfast

Cheese Broccoli Chaffles

Preparation Time: 5 minutes

Cooking Time: 16 minutes

Servings: 4

Ingredients:

- 1/2 cup Cooked broccoli, chopped finely
- 2 organic eggs, beaten
- 1/2 cup Cheddar cheese, shredded
- 1/2 cup Mozzarella cheese, shredded
- 2 tablespoons Parmesan cheese, grated
- 1/2 teaspoon onion powder

Directions:

1. Preheat a Chaffle iron and then grease it.
2. In a bowl, place all Ingredients and mix until well merged.
3. Set half of the mixture into preheated Chaffle iron and Cooking for about 4 minutes or until golden brown.
4. Repeat with the remaining mixture.
5. Serve warm.

Nutrition:

Calories: 112

Net Carb: 1.2g

Fat: 8.1g

Saturated Fat: 4.3g

Carbohydrates: 1.59

Sugar: 0.5g

Protein: 8.

Bacon and Ham Chaffle

Preparation Time: 5 minutes

Cooking Time: 5 minutes

Servings: 2

Ingredients:

- 3 egg
- 1/2 cup grated Cheddar cheese
- 1 Tbsp. almond flour
- 1/2 tsp. baking powder

For the toppings:

- 4 strips Cooked bacon
- 2 pieces Bibb lettuce
- 2 slices preferable ham
- 2 slices tomato

Directions:

1. Turn on Chaffle maker to heat and oil it with Cooking spray.
2. Combine all chaffle components in a small bowl.
3. Add around 1/4 of total batter to Chaffle maker and spread to fill the edges. Close and Cooking for 4 minutes.
4. Remove and let it cool on a rack.
5. Repeat for the second chaffle.

6. Top one chaffle with a tomato slice, a piece of lettuce, and bacon strips, and then cover it with second chaffle.

7. Plate and enjoy.

Nutrition

Carbs: 5g

Fat: 60 g

Protein: 31 g

Calories: 631

Ham and Jalapenos Chaffle

Preparation Time: 5 minutes

Cooking Time: 9 minutes

Servings: 3

Ingredients:

- 2 Tbsp. cheddar cheese, finely grated
- 2 large eggs
- 1/2 jalapeno pepper, finely grated
- 2 ounces ham steak
- 1 medium scallion
- 2 tsp. coconut flour

Directions:

1. Set your Chaffle iron with Cooking spray and heat for 3 minutes.
2. Pour 1/4 of the batter mixture into the Chaffle iron.
3. Cooking for 3 minutes, until crispy around the edges.
4. Remove the Chaffles from the heat and repeat until all the batter is finished.
5. Once done, allow them to cool to room temperature and enjoy.
6. Shred the cheddar cheese using a fine grater.
7. Deseed the jalapeno and grate using the same grater.

8. Finely chop the scallion and ham.

9. Serve!

Nutrition

Calories: 120

Fats: 10 g

Carbs: 2 g

Protein: 12

Crispy Bagel Chaffle

Preparation Time: 15 minutes

Cooking Time: 30 minutes

Servings: 1

Ingredients:

- 2 eggs
- 2 cup parmesan cheese
- 1 tsp. bagel seasoning
- 1/2 cup mozzarella cheese
- 2 teaspoons almond flour

Directions:

1. Turn on Chaffle maker to heat and oil it with Cooking spray.
2. Evenly sprinkle half of cheeses to a griddle and let them melt. Then toast for 30 seconds and leave them wait for batter.
3. Whisk eggs, other half of cheeses, almond flour, and bagel seasoning in a small bowl.
4. Pour batter into the Chaffle, Cooking for minutes.
5. Let cool for 2-3 minutes before serving.

Nutrition:

Carbs: g

Fat: 20 g

Protein: 21 g

Calories: 28 7

Sausage and Veggies Chaffles

Preparation Time: 5 minutes

Cooking Time: 20 minutes

Servings: 4

Ingredients:

- 1/3 cup unsweetened almond milk
- 4 medium organic eggs
- 2 tablespoons gluten-free breakfast sausage, cut into slices
- 2 tablespoons broccoli florets, chopped
- 2 tablespoons bell peppers, seeded and chopped
- 2 tablespoons Mozzarella cheese, shredded

Directions:

1. Preheat a Chaffle iron and then grease it.
2. In a medium bowl, place the almond milk and eggs and beat well.
3. Place the remaining Ingredients: and stir to combine well.
4. Place 1/4 of the mixture into preheated Chaffle iron and Cooking for about 5 minutes or until golden brown.
5. Repeat with the remaining mixture.
6. Serve warm.

Nutrition:

Calories: 13 2

Net Carb: 1.2 g

Fat: 9.2 g

Saturated Fat: 3.5g

Carbohydrates: 1

Sugar: 0.5 g

Protein: 11.1g

Bacon and Serrano Pepper Chaffles

Preparation Time: 5 minutes

Cooking Time: 10 minutes

Servings: 2

Ingredients:

- 1 organic egg, beaten
- 1/2 cup Cheddar cheese, shredded
- 1/4 cup fresh broccoli, chopped
- 1 tablespoon almond flour
- 1/4 teaspoon garlic powder

Directions:

1. Preheat a mini Chaffle iron and then grease It.
2. In a bowl, place all Ingredients: and mix until well merged.
3. Set half of the mixture into preheated Chaffle iron and Cooking for about 4 minutes or until golden brown.
4. Repeat with the remaining mixture.
5. Serve warm.

Nutrition:

Calories: 17 3

Net Carb: 1.5 g

Fat: 13.5 g

Saturated Fat: 8g

Carbohydrates: 2.2 g

Sugar: 0.7g

Protein: 10.2 g

Garlic Powder Chaffles

Preparation Time: 5 minutes

Cooking Time: 8 minutes

Servings: 2

Ingredients:

- 1 organic egg, beaten
- 1/2 cup Monterrey Jack cheese, shredded
- 1 teaspoon coconut flour
- Pinch of garlic powder

Directions:

1. Preheat a mini Chaffle iron and then grease it.
2. In a bowl, merge all the Ingredients: and beat until well merged.
3. Set half of the mixture into preheated Chaffle iron and Cooking for about 4 minutes or until golden brown.
4. Repeat with the remaining mixture.
5. Serve warm.

Nutrition:

Calories: 147

Net Carb: 1.

Fat: 1 1.3 g

Saturated Fat: 6.8g

Carbohydrates: 2.1g

Sugar: 0.2g

Protein: 9g

Bacon Chaffle Omelets

Preparation Time: 5 minutes

Cooking Time: 10 minutes

Servings: 2

Ingredients:

- 2 slices bacon, raw
- 1egg
- 1 tsp. maple extract, optional
- 1 tsp. all spices

Directions:

1. Put the bacon slices in a blender and tum. , it on.
2. Once ground up, add in the egg and all spices. Go on blending until liquefied.
3. Heat your Chaffle maker on the highest setting and spray with non-stick Cooking spray.
4. Pour half the omelets into the Chaffle maker and Cooking for 5 minutes max.
5. Remove the crispy omelet and repeat the same steps wit rest batter.
6. Enjoy warm

Nutrition:

Calories: 59

Fats: 4.4 g

Carbs: 1 g

Protein: 5 g

Bacon Chaffles For Couples

Preparation Time: 5 minutes

Cooking Time: 5 minutes

Servings: 2

Ingredients:

- 2 eggs
- 1/2 cup cheddar cheese
- 1/2 cup mozzarella cheese
- 1/4 tsp. baking powder
- 1/2 Tbsp. almond flour
- 1 Tbsp. butter, for Chaffle maker

For the filling:

- 1/4 cup bacon, chopped
- 2 Tbsp. green onions, chopped

Directions:

1. Turn on Chaffle maker to heat and oil it with Cooking spray.
2. Add eggs, mozzarella, cheddar, almond flour, and baking powder to a blender and pulse 10 times, so cheese is still chunky.
3. Add bacon and green onions. Pulse 2-times to combine.

4. Attach one half of the batter to the Chaffle maker and Cooking for 3 minutes, until golden brown.
5. Repeat with remaining batter.
6. Add your toppings and serve hot.

Nutrition:

Carbs: 3 g

Fat: 3 8 g

Protein: 23 g

Calories: 446

Yeast Chaffles

Preparation Time: 5 minutes

Cooking Time: 5 minutes

Servings: 2

Ingredients:

- 2 cups almond milk
- 1 (0.25 ounce) package active dry yeast
- 1/2 cup warm water
- 1/2 cup butter, melted
- 1 teaspoon salt
- 1 teaspoon sugar substitute
- 1/2 cup mozzarella cheese, shredded
- 3 cups almond flour
- 2 eggs, slightly beaten
- 1/2 teaspoon baking soda

Directions:

1. Warm the almond milk in a small saucepan until it bubbles, then remove from heat. In a bowl, dissolve yeast in water. Let stand until creamy, about 10 minutes.
2. In a large bowl, combine almond milk, yeast mixture, butter, salt, sugar substitute and flour. Add mozzarella cheese and stir well.

3. Mix thoroughly with rotary or electric mixer until batter is smooth. Secure and let stand at room temperature overnight.
4. The next morning, stir beaten eggs and baking soda into the batter; beat well.
5. Set preheated Chaffle iron with non-stick Cooking spray. Pour mix onto hot Chaffle iron. Cooking until golden brown.

Nutrition:

Calories 434

Total Fat 29.3 g

Cholesterol 109 mg,

Sodium 661 mg,

Total Carbohydrate 9.8 g,

Protein 16.8 g

Cheddar, Whipping Cream & Sun Butter Chaffles

Preparation Time: 5 minutes

Cooking Time: 18 minutes

Servings: 2

Ingredients:

- 1/2 cup cheddar cheese, shredded
- 1 organic egg
- 1 organic egg white
- 2 tablespoons heavy whipping cream
- 1 tablespoon sugar-free sun butter
- 2 tablespoons coconut flour
- 3 tablespoons Erythritol
- 1/4 teaspoon organic vanilla extract
- 1/8 teaspoon organic baking powder

Directions:

1. Preheat a mini Chaffle iron and then grease it.
2. In a medium bowl, merge all ingredients and with a fork, mix until well combined.
3. Divide the mixture into 6 portions.
4. Place 1 portion of the mixture into preheated Chaffle iron and cook for about 2-3 minutes or until golden brown.

5. Repeat with the remaining mixture.

6. Serve warm.

Nutrition:

Calories: 95

Net Carb: 1.4g

Fat: 7.3g

Carbohydrates: 2.6g

Dietary Fiber: 1.2g

Sugar: 0.4g

Protein: 5g

Spring Onion Buns

Preparation Time: 10 minutes

Cooking Time: 30 minutes

Servings: 6

Ingredients

- 3 eggs, separated
- 3 1/2 oz. cream cheese
- 1 tsp. stevia
- 1/2 tsp. baking powder
- Salt to taste
- For the filling
- 1 egg, hard-boiled, chopped
- 2 sprigs spring onions, chopped

Directions

1. Combine egg yolks with stevia, cream cheese, baking powder, and salt.
2. Whisk egg whites until foamy.
3. Merge the egg whites into the yolk mixture.
4. Pour the dough into greased muffin cups filling 1/2 of the cup.
5. Combine spring onions with chopped egg and add this filling to muffin cups.
6. Pour more dough into the cups.
7. Bake at 300F for 30 minutes.

8. Serve.

Nutrition:

Calories: 81

Fat: 6.7g

Carb: 1.1g

Protein: 4.2g

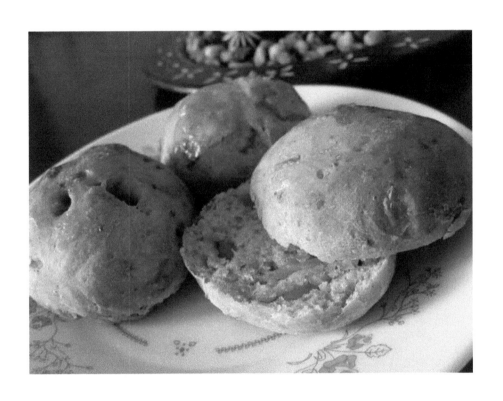

Lemon and Coconut Cookies

Preparation Time: 10 minutes

Cooking Time: 15 minutes

Servings: 24

Ingredients

- 1 cup butter, softened
- 1/2 cup granulated sugar substitute
- 1 1/2 cups coconut flour
- 4 eggs
- 1/2 tsp. salt
- 1/4 cup chopped almonds
- 2 tsp. lemon extract

Directions

1. Preheat the oven to 375F.
2. Line two cookies sheets with parchment paper.
3. In a bowl, combine the sugar substitute, lemon extract, salt, and butter and beat well together.
4. Attach the eggs one at a time, beating well after each addition.
5. Stir in the coconut flour.
6. Drop spoon fuls of the mix onto the prepared sheets, flatten with a fork.
7. Top with a sprinkle of chopped almonds and bake for 12 to 15 minutes.

8. Turn the cookies after 8 minutes to brown evenly.

9. Remove and serve.

Nutrition:

Calories: 118

Fat: 9.6g

Carb: 4.7g

Protein: 2.2g

Sandwich Rolls

Preparation Time: 10 minutes

Cooking Time: 14 minutes

Servings: 6

Ingredients

- 1 cup almond flour
- 1/4 tsp. baking soda
- 1/2 tsp. salt
- 4 Tbsp. unsalted butter, melted
- 4 eggs
- 2 Tbsp. almond milk
- 2 Tbsp. topping (poppy seeds or sesame seeds)

Directions

1. Preheat the oven to 425F.
2. Merge the almond flour, baking soda, and salt in a bowl and blend well.
3. Add the wet ingredients to the bowl and mix well.
4. Divide the batter among a muffin top baking pan. Sprinkle with topping.
5. Bake for 12 to 14 minutes.
6. Cool and serve.

Nutrition:

Calories: 143

Fat: 13g

Carb: 1g

Protein: 5g

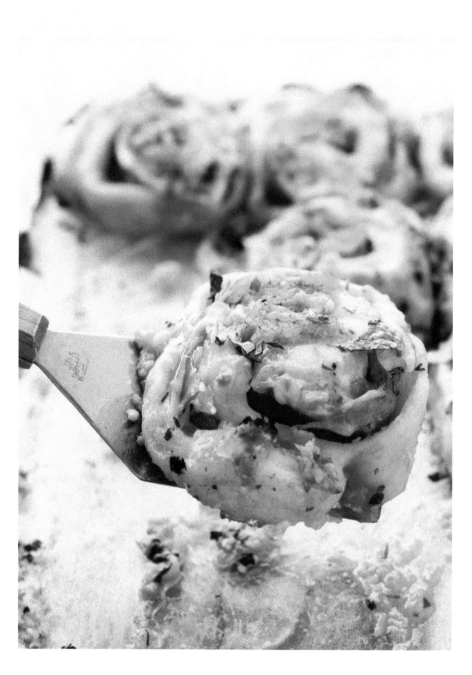

Ham and Cheese Rolls

Preparation Time: 10 minutes

Cooking Time: 18 minutes

Servings: 6

Ingredients

- 1/2 cup cheddar cheese, shredded
- 1 cup deli ham, diced
- 3/4 cup mozzarella cheese, shredded
- 2 eggs
- 1/2 cup parmesan cheese, grated

Directions

1. Preheat the oven to 375F. Line a flat sheet with baking paper.
2. Blend the diced ham, eggs, mozzarella, parmesan and cheddar cheese in a glass dish until mixed.
3. Set the batter into 6 equal parts and create mounds. Transfer to the prepared flat sheet.
4. Bake in the oven for 18 minutes.
5. Enjoy.

Nutrition:

Calories: 198

Fat: 13g

Carb: 3g

Protein: 17g

Pumpkin Pecan Chaffles

Preparation Time: 10 minutes

Cooking Time: 10 minutes

Servings: 2

Ingredients:

- 1 egg
- 1/2 cup mozzarella cheese grated
- 1 Tbsp. pumpkin puree
- 1/2 tsp. pumpkin spice
- 1 tsp. Erythritol low carb sweetener
- 2 Tbsp. almond flour
- 2 Tbsp. pecans, toasted chopped
- 1 cup heavy whipped cream
- 1/4 cup low carb caramel sauce

Directions:

1. Turn on Chaffle maker to heat and oil it with Cooking spray. In a bowl, beat egg.
2. Mix in mozzarella, pumpkin, flour, pumpkin spice, and Erythritol. Stir in pecan pieces.
3. Spoon one half of the batter into Chaffle maker and spread evenly. Close and Cooking for 5 minutes.
4. Remove Cooked Chaffles to a plate. Repeat with remaining batter.

5. Serve with pecans, whipped cream, and low carb caramel sauce.

Nutrition:

Carbs 4 g

Fat 17 g

Protein 11 g

Calories 210

Italian Cream Chaffle Sandwich-Cake

Preparation Time: 5 minutes

Cooking Time: 8 minutes

Servings: 2

Ingredients:

- 4 oz. cream cheese, softened, at room temperature
- 4 eggs
- 1 Tbsp. melted butter
- 1 tsp. vanilla extract
- 1/2 tsp. cinnamon
- 1 Tbsp. monk fruit sweetener
- 4 Tbsp. coconut flour
- 1 Tbsp. almond flour
- 11/2 teaspoons baking powder
- 1 Tbsp. coconut, shredded and unsweetened
- 1 Tbsp. walnuts, chopped

For the Italian Cream Frosting:

- 2 oz. cream cheese, softened, at room temperature
- 2 Tbsp. butter room temp
- 2 Tbsp. monk fruit sweetener
- 1/2 tsp. vanilla

Directions:

1. Combine cream cheese, eggs, melted butter, vanilla, sweetener, flours, and baking powder in a blender. Add walnuts and coconut to the mixture.
2. Blend to get a creamy mixture.
3. Turn on Chaffle maker to heat and oil it with Cooking spray.
4. Add enough batter to fill Chaffle maker. Cooking for 2-3 minutes, until chaffles are done. Remove and let them cool.
5. Mix all frosting ingredients in another bowl. Stir until smooth and creamy. Frost the chaffles once they have cooled.
6. Top with cream and more nuts.

Nutrition:

Carbs 31 g

Fat 2 g

Protein 5 g

Calories 168

Chocolate Cherry Chaffles

Preparation Time: 5 minutes

Cooking Time: 5 minutes

Servings: 1

Ingredients:

- 1 Tbsp. almond flour
- 1 Tbsp. cocoa powder
- 1 Tbsp. sugar free sweetener
- 1/2 tsp. baking powder
- 1 whole egg
- 1/2 cup mozzarella cheese shredded
- 2 Tbsp. heavy whipping cream whipped
- 2 Tbsp. sugar free cherry pie filling
- 1 Tbsp. chocolate chips

Directions:

1. Turn on Chaffle maker to heat and oil it with Cooking spray. Mix all dry components in a bowl.
2. Add egg and mix well.
3. Add cheese and stir again.
4. Spoon batter into Chaffle maker and close. Cooking for 5 minutes, until done.
5. Top with whipping cream, cherries, and chocolate chips.

Nutrition:

Carbs 6 g

Fat 1 g

Protein 1 g

Calories 130

Banana Nut Chaffle

Preparation Time: 10 minutes

Cooking Time: 5 minutes

Servings: 1

Ingredients:

- 1 egg
- 1 Tbsp. cream cheese, softened and room temp
- 1 Tbsp. sugar-free cheesecake pudding
- 1/2 cup mozzarella cheese
- 1 Tbsp. monk fruit confectioners sweetener
- 1/4 tsp. vanilla extract
- 1/4 tsp. banana extract
- toppings of choice

Directions:

1. Turn on Chaffle maker to heat and oil it with Cooking spray. Beat egg in a small bowl.
2. Attach remaining ingredients and mix until well incorporated.
3. Add one half of the batter to Chaffle maker and Cooking for 4 minutes, until golden brown. Remove chaffle and add the other half of the batter.
4. Top with your optional toppings and serve warm!

Nutrition:

Carbs 2 g

Fat 7 g

Protein 8 g

Calories 119

Belgium Chaffles

Preparation Time: 5 minutes

Cooking Time: 6 minutes

Servings: 1

Ingredients:

- 2 eggs
- 1 cup Reduced-fat Cheddar cheese, shredded

Directions:

1. Turn on Chaffle maker to heat and oil it with Cooking spray.
2. Whisk eggs in a bowl, add cheese. Stir until well-combined.
3. Pour mixture into Chaffle maker and Cooking for 6 minutes until done. Let it cool a little too crisp before serving.

Nutrition:

Carbs 2 g

Fat 33 g

Protein 44 g

Calories 460

Bacon Chaffles

Preparation Time: 5 minutes

Cooking Time: 5 minutes

Servings: 2

Ingredients:

- 2 eggs
- 1/2 cup cheddar cheese
- 1/2 cup mozzarella cheese
- 1/4 tsp. baking powder
- 1/2 Tbsp. almond flour
- 1 Tbsp. butter, for Chaffle maker

For the Filling:

- 1/4 cup bacon, chopped
- 2 Tbsp. green onions, chopped

Directions:

1. Turn on Chaffle maker to heat and oil it with Cooking spray.
2. Add eggs, mozzarella, cheddar, almond flour, and baking powder to a blender and pulse 10 times, so cheese is still chunky.
3. Add bacon and green onions. Pulse 2-3 times to combine.

4. Attach one half of the batter to the Chaffle maker and Cooking for 3 minutes, until golden brown.
5. Repeat with remaining batter.
6. Add your toppings and serve hot.

Nutrition:

Carbs 3 g

Fat 38 g

Protein 23 g

Calories 446

Chaffle Egg Sandwich

Preparation Time: 5 minutes

Cooking Time: 10 minutes

Servings: 2

Ingredients:

- 2 slice cheddar cheese
- 1 egg simple omelet

Directions:

1. Prepare your oven on 400 F.
2. Arrange egg omelet and cheese slice between chaffles.
3. Bake in the warmth oven for about 4-5 minutes until cheese is melted.
4. Once the cheese is melted, detach from the oven.
5. Serve and enjoy!

Nutrition:

Protein: 144

Fat: 337

Carbohydrates: 14

Chaffle Minutesi Sandwich

Preparation Time: 5 minutes

Cooking Time: 10 minutes

Servings: 2

Ingredients:

- 1 large egg
- 1/8 cup almond flour
- 1/2 tsp. garlic powder
- 3/4 tsp. baking powder
- 1/2 cup shredded cheese

Sandwich Filling:

- 2 slices deli ham
- 2 slices tomatoes
- 1 slice cheddar cheese

Directions:

1. Grease your square Chaffle maker and preheat it on medium heat.
2. Mix together chaffle ingredients in a mixing bowl until well combined.
3. Pour batter into a square Chaffle and make two chaffles.
4. Once chaffles are Cooked, remove from the maker.

5. For a sandwich, arrange deli ham, tomato slice and cheddar cheese between two chaffles.
6. Cut sandwich from the center.
7. Serve and enjoy!

Nutrition:

Calories 208

Fat 13.5g

Carbohydrate 0.7g

Protein 8.2g

Sugars 0.6g

Chaffle Cheese Sandwich

Preparation Time: 5 minutes

Cooking Time: 10 minutes

Servings: 1

Ingredients:

- 2 square keto chaffle
- 2 slice cheddar cheese
- 2 lettuce leaves

Directions:

1. Prepare your oven on 400 F.
2. Arrange lettuce leave and cheese slice between chaffles.
3. Bake in the warmth oven for about 4-5 minutes until cheese is melted.
4. Once the cheese is melted, detach from the oven.
5. Serve and enjoy!

Nutrition:

Calories 208

Fat 13.5g

Carbohydrate 0.7g

Protein 8.2g

Sugars 0.6g

Spicy Chicken Zinger Chaffle

Preparation Time: 5 minutes

Cooking Time: 15 minutes

Servings: 2

Ingredients:

- 1 chicken breast, cut into 2 pieces
- 1/2 cup coconut flour
- 1/4 cup finely grated Parmesan
- 1 tsp. paprika
- 1/2 tsp. garlic powder
- 1/2 tsp. onion powder
- 1 tsp. salt and pepper
- 1 tsp. chili powder
- 1 egg beaten
- Avocado oil for frying Lettuce leaves
- BBQ sauce

Chaffle Ingredients:

- 4 oz. cheese
- 2 whole eggs
- 2 oz. almond flour
- 1/4 cup almond flour
- 1 tsp. baking powder

Directions:

1. Mix together chaffle ingredients in a bowl.
2. Pour the chaffle batter in preheated greased square chaffle maker.
3. Cooking chaffles for about 2-minutes until Cooked through.
4. Make square chaffles from this batter.
5. Meanwhile mix together coconut flour, parmesan, paprika, garlic powder, onion powder salt and pepper in a bowl.
6. Dip chicken first in coconut flour mixture then in beaten egg.
7. Heat avocado oil in a skillet and Cooking chicken from both sides. until lightly brown and Cooked
8. Set chicken zinger between two chaffles with lettuce and BBQ sauce.
9. Enjoy!

Nutrition:

Calories 208

Fat 13.5g

Carbohydrate 0.7g

Protein 8.2g

Sugars 0.6g

Peanut Butter and Jelly Sammich Chaffle

Preparation Time: 20 minutes

Cooking Time: 30 minutes

Servings: 2

Ingredients:

For Chaffle:

- Egg: 2
- Mozzarella: 1/4 cup
- Vanilla extract: 1 tbsp.
- Coconut flour: 2 tbsp.
- Baking powder: 1/4 tsp.
- Cinnamon powder: 1 tsp.
- Swerve sweetener: 1 tbsp.
- For Blueberry Compote:
- Blueberries: 1 cup
- Lemon zest: 1/2 tsp.
- Lemon juice: 1 tsp.
- Xanthan gum: 1/8 tsp.
- Water: 2 tbsp.
- Swerve sweetener: 1 tbsp.

Directions:

1. For the blueberry compote, add all the ingredients except xanthan gum to a small pan
2. Mix them all and boil
3. Set the heat and simmer for 8-10 minutes; the sauce will initiate to thicken
4. Add xanthan gum now and stir
5. Now remove the pan from the stove and allow the mixture to cool down
6. Put in refrigerator
7. Preheat a mini Chaffle maker if needed and grease it
8. In a mixing bowl, add all the chaffle ingredients and mix well
9. Pour the mixture to the lower plate of the Chaffle maker and spread it evenly to cover the plate properly
10. Close the lid
11. Cooking for at least 4 minutes to get the desired crunch
12. Remove the chaffle from the heat and keep aside
13. Make as many chaffles as your mixture and Chaffle maker allow
14. Serve with the blueberry and enjoy!

Nutrition:

Calories: 175

Total Fat: 15g

Carbs: 8g

Net Carbs: 5g

Fiber: 3g

Protein: 6g

Peanut Butter Cup Chaffles

Preparation Time: 5 minutes

Cooking Time: 15 minutes

Servings: 1

Ingredients:

For the chaffle:

- Eggs: 1
- Mozzarella cheese: 1/2 cup shredded
- Cocoa powder: 2 tbsp.
- Espresso powder: 1/4 tsp.
- Sugar free chocolate chips: 1 tbsp.

For the filling:

- Peanut butter: 3 tbsp.
- Butter: 1 tbsp.
- Powdered sweetener: 2 tbsp.

Direction:

1. Add all the chaffle ingredients in a bowl and whisk
2. Preheat your mini Chaffle iron if needed and grease it
3. Cooking your mixture in the mini Chaffle iron for at least 4 minutes
4. Make two chaffles
5. Mix the filling ingredients together.

6. When chaffles cool down, spread peanut butter on them to make a sandwich

Nutrition:

Calories: 448

Total Fat: 34g

Carbs: 17g

Net Carbs: 10g

Fiber: 7g

Protein: 24g

Chocolaty Chaffles

Preparation Time: 5 minutes

Cooking Time: 15 minutes

Servings: 1

Ingredients:

- Eggs: 1
- Mozzarella cheese: 1/2 cup shredded
- Cocoa powder: 2 tbsp.
- Espresso powder: 1/4 tsp.
- Sugar free chocolate chips: 1 tbsp.

Directions:

1. Add all the chaffle ingredients in a bowl and whisk
2. Preheat your mini Chaffle iron if needed and grease it
3. Cooking your mixture in the mini Chaffle iron for at least 4 minutes
4. Make as many chaffles as you can

Nutrition:

Calories: 258

Total Fat: 23g

Carbs: 12g

Net Carbs: 6g

Fiber: 6g

Protein: 5g

Mc Griddle Chaffle

Preparation Time: 5 minutes

Cooking Time: 10 minutes

Servings: 2

Ingredients:

- Egg: 2
- Mozzarella cheese: 11/2 cup (shredded)
- Maple Syrup: 2 tbsp. (sugar-free)
- Sausage patty: 2
- American cheese: 2 slices
- Swerve/Monkfruit: 2 tbsp.

Directions:

1. Preheat a mini Chaffle maker if needed and grease it
2. In a mixing bowl, beat eggs and add shredded Mozzarella cheese, Swerve/Monkfruit, and maple syrup
3. Merge them all well and pour the mixture to the lower plate of the Chaffle maker
4. Close the lid
5. Cooking for at least 4 minutes to get the desired crunch
6. Remove the chaffle from the heat

7. sausage patty by following the instruction given on the packaging
8. Place a cheese slice on the patty immediately when removing from heat
9. Take two chaffles and put sausage patty and cheese in between
10. Make as many chaffles as your mixture and Chaffle maker allow
11. Serve hot and enjoy!

Nutrition:

Calories: 231

Total Fat: 20g

Carbs: 8g

Net Carbs: 6g

Fiber: 2g

Protein: 9g

Cinnamon Swirl Chaffles

Preparation Time: 5 minutes

Cooking Time: 10 minutes

Servings: 2

Ingredients:

For Chaffle:

- Egg: 2
- Cream Cheese: 2 oz. softened
- Almond flour: 2 tbsp.
- Vanilla Extract: 2 tsp.
- Cinnamon: 2 tsp.
- Vanilla extract: 2 tsp.
- Splenda: 2 tbsp.

For Icing:

- Cream cheese: 2 oz. softened
- Splenda: 2 tbsp.
- Vanilla: 1 tsp.
- Butter: 2 tbsp. unsalted butter

For Cinnamon Drizzle:

- Splenda: 2 tbsp.
- Butter: 1 tbsp.
- Cinnamon: 2 tsp.

Directions:

1. Preheat the Chaffle maker
2. Grease it lightly
3. Mix all the chaffle ingredients together
4. Pour the mixture to the Chaffle maker
5. Cooking for around 4 minutes or till chaffles become crispy
6. Keep them aside when done
7. In a small bowl, mix the ingredients of icing and cinnamon drizzle
8. Heat it in a microwave for about 10 seconds to gain a soft uniformity
9. Whirl on cooled chaffles and enjoy!

Nutrition:

Calories: 323

Total Fat: 27g

Carbs: 8g

Net Carbs: 3g;

Fiber: 5g

Protein: 15g

Raspberries Chaffle

Preparation time: 15 minutes

Cooking Time: 15 Minutes

Servings: 1

Ingredients:

- 1 egg white
- 1/4 cup jack cheese, shredded
- 1/4 cup cheddar cheese, shredded
- 1 tsp. coconut flour
- 1/4 tsp. baking powder
- 1/2 tsp. stevia

For Topping

- 4 oz. raspberries
- 2 tbsps. coconut flour
- 2 oz. unsweetened raspberry sauce

Directions:

1. Switch on your round Chaffle Maker and grease it with cooking spray once it is hot.
2. Mix together all chaffle ingredients in a bowl and combine with a fork.
3. Pour chaffle batter in a preheated maker and close the lid.

4. Roll the taco chaffle around using a kitchen roller, set it aside and allow it to set for a few minutes.
5. Once the taco chaffle is set, remove from the roller.
6. Dip raspberries in sauce and arrange on taco chaffle.
7. Drizzle coconut flour on top.
8. Enjoy raspberries taco chaffle with keto coffee.

Nutrition:

Calories: 386

Total Fat: 37g

Carbs: 13g

Net Carbs: 8g;

Fiber: 5g

Protein: 5g

Garlic and Parsley Chaffles

Preparation time: 10 minutes

Cooking Time: 5 Minutes

Servings: 1

Ingredients:

- 1 large egg
- 1/4 cup cheese Mozzarella
- 1 tsp. coconut flour
- 1/4 tsp. baking powder
- 1/2 tsp. garlic powder
- 1 tbsp. minute sced parsley

For Serving

- 1 Poach egg
- 4 oz. smoked salmon

Directions:

1. Switch on your Dash Chaffle maker and let it preheat.
2. Grease Chaffle maker with cooking spray.
3. Mix together egg, mozzarella, coconut flour, and baking powder, and garlic powder, parsley to a mixing bowl until combined well.
4. Pour batter in circle chaffle maker.
5. Close the lid.

6. Cooking for about 2-3 minutes or until the Chaffles is Cooked.
7. Serve with smoked salmon and poached egg.
8. Enjoy!

Nutrition:

Calories: 757

Total Fat: 38g

Carbs: 17g

Net Carbs: 11g

Fiber: 6g

Protein: 29g

Scrambled Eggs and a Spring Onion Chaffle

Preparation time: 10 minutes

Cooking Time: 7-9 Minutes

Servings: 4

Ingredients:

Batter

- 4 eggs
- 2 cups grated Mozzarella cheese
- 2 spring onions, finely chopped
- Salt and pepper to taste
- 1/2 teaspoon dried garlic powder
- 2 tablespoons almond flour
- 2 tablespoons coconut flour

Other

- 2 tablespoons butter for brushing the Chaffle maker
- 6-8 eggs
- Salt and pepper
- 1 teaspoon Italian spice mix
- 1 tablespoon olive oil
- 1 tablespoon freshly chopped parsley

Directions:

1. Preheat the Chaffle maker.

71

2. Whisk the eggs into a bowl and add the grated cheese.
3. Mix until just combined, then add the chopped spring onions and season with salt and pepper and dried garlic powder.
4. Stir in the almond flour and mix until everything is combined.
5. Brush the heated Chaffle maker with butter and add a few tablespoons of the batter.
6. Close the lid and Cooking for about 7–8 minutes depending on your Chaffle maker.
7. While the chaffles are Cooking, the scrambled eggs by whisking the eggs in a bowl until frothy, about 2 minutes. Flavor with salt and black pepper to taste and add the Italian spice mix. Whisk to blend in the spices.
8. Warm the oil in a non-stick pan over medium heat.
9. Pour the eggs in the pan and Cooking until eggs are set to your liking.
10. Serve each chaffle and top with some scrambled eggs. Top with freshly chopped parsley.

Nutrition:

Calories: 165

Total Fat: 15

Carbs: 4g

Net Carbs: 2g

Fiber: 2g

Protein: 6g

Egg and Cheddar Cheese Chaffle

Preparation time: 10 minutes

Cooking Time: 7-9 Minutes

Servings: 4

Ingredients:

Batter

- 4 eggs
- 2 cups shredded white cheddar cheese
- Salt and pepper to taste

Other

- 2 tablespoons butter for brushing the Chaffle maker
- 4 large eggs
- 2 tablespoons olive oil

Directions:

1. Preheat the Chaffle maker.
2. Beat the eggs into a bowl and whisk them with a fork.
3. Stir in the grated cheddar cheese and season with salt and pepper.
4. Brush the heated Chaffle maker with butter and add a few tablespoons of the batter.
5. Close the lid and Cooking for about 7–8 minutes depending on your Chaffle maker.

74

6. While chaffles are Cooking, Cooking the eggs.
7. Set the oil in a large non-stick pan that has a lid over medium-low heat for 2-3 minutes
8. Crack an egg in a small ramekin and gently add it to the pan. Repeat the same way for the other 3 eggs.
9. Cover and let Cooking for 2 to 2 1/2 minutes for set eggs but with runny yolks.
10. Remove from heat.
11. To serve, place a chaffle on each plate and top with an egg. Flavor with salt and black pepper to taste.

Nutrition:

Calories: 74

Total Fat: 7g

Carbs: 1g

Net Carbs: 0g

Fiber: 0g

Protein: 3g

Chili Chaffle

Preparation time: 10 minutes

Cooking Time: 7-9 Minutes

Servings: 4

Ingredients:

Batter

- 4 eggs
- 1/2 cup grated parmesan cheese
- 11/2 cups grated yellow cheddar cheese
- 1 hot red chili pepper
- Salt and pepper to taste
- 1/2 teaspoon dried garlic powder
- 1 teaspoon dried basil
- 2 tablespoons almond flour

Other

- 2 tablespoons olive oil for brushing the Chaffle maker

Directions:

1. Preheat the Chaffle maker.
2. Whisk the eggs into a bowl and add the grated parmesan and cheddar cheese.

3. Mix until just combined and add the chopped chili pepper. Season with salt and pepper, dried garlic powder and dried basil. Stir in the almond flour.
4. Mix until everything is combined.
5. Brush the heated Chaffle maker with olive oil and add a few tablespoons of the batter.
6. Close the lid and Cooking for about 7–8 minutes depending on your Chaffle maker.

Nutrition:

Calories: 859

Total Fat: 73g

Carbs: 8g

Net Carbs: 8g

Fiber: 0g

Protein: 41g

Simple Savory Chaffle

Preparation time: 10 minutes

Cooking Time: 7–9 Minutes

Servings: 4

Ingredients:

Batter

- 4 eggs
- 1 cup grated Mozzarella cheese
- 1 cup grated provolone cheese
- 1/2 cup almond flour
- 2 tablespoons coconut flour
- 21/2 teaspoons baking powder
- Salt and pepper to taste

Other

- 2 tablespoons butter to brush the Chaffle maker

Directions:

1. Preheat the Chaffle maker.
2. Add the grated Mozzarella and provolone cheese to a bowl and mix.
3. Add the almond and coconut flour and baking powder and season with salt and pepper.
4. Mix with a wire whisk and crack in the eggs.
5. Stir everything together until batter forms.

6. Brush the heated Chaffle maker with butter and add a few tablespoons of the batter.
7. Close the lid and Cooking for about 8 minutes depending on your Chaffle maker.
8. Serve and enjoy.

Nutrition:

Calories: 248

Total Fat: 18g

Carbs: 11g

Net Carbs: 7g

Fiber: 5g

Protein: 14g

Pizza Chaffles

Preparation time: 10 minutes

Cooking Time: 7-9 Minutes

Servings: 4

Ingredients:

Batter

- 4 eggs
- 11/2 cups grated Mozzarella cheese
- 1/2 cup grated parmesan cheese
- 2 tablespoons tomato sauce
- 1/4 cup almond flour
- 11/2 teaspoons baking powder
- Salt and pepper to taste
- 1 teaspoon dried oregano
- 1/4 cup sliced salami

Other

- 2 tablespoons olive oil for brushing the Chaffle maker
- 1/4 cup tomato sauce for serving

Directions:

1. Preheat the Chaffle maker.
2. Add the grated Mozzarella and grated parmesan to a bowl and mix.

3. Add the almond flour and baking powder and season with salt and pepper and dried oregano.
4. Merge with a wooden spoon or wire whisk and crack in the eggs.
5. Stir everything together until batter forms.
6. Stir in the chopped salami.
7. Brush the heated Chaffle maker with olive oil and add a few tablespoons of the batter.
8. Close the lid and Cooking for about 7-minutes depending on your Chaffle maker.
9. Serve with extra tomato sauce on top and enjoy.

Nutrition:

Calories: 583

Total Fat: 54g

Carbs: 7g

Net Carbs: 7g

Fiber: 0g

Protein: 19g

Simple Chaffle

Preparation time: 10 minutes

Cooking Time: 5 minutes

Servings: 4

Ingredients:

- 1 cup egg whites
- 1 cup cheddar cheese, shredded
- 1/4 cup almond flour
- 1/4 cup heavy cream
- 4 oz. raspberries
- 4 oz. strawberries.
- 1 oz. keto chocolate flakes
- 1 oz. feta cheese.

Directions:

1. Preheat your square Chaffle maker and grease with cooking spray.
2. Whisk egg white in a bowl with flour.
3. Add shredded cheese to the egg whites and flour mixture and mix well.
4. Add cream and cheese to the egg mixture.
5. Pour Chaffles batter in a Chaffle maker and close the lid.
6. Cooking chaffles for about 4 minutes until crispy and brown.

7. Carefully remove chaffles from the maker.
8. Serve with berries, cheese, and chocolate on top.
9. Enjoy!

Nutrition:

Calories: 254

Total Fat: 19g

Carbs: 11g

Net Carbs: 7g

Fiber: 4g

Protein: 11g

Chaffles Breakfast Bowl

Preparation Time: 15 minutes

Cooking Time: 5 minutes

Servings: 2

Ingredients:

- 1 egg
- 1/2 cup cheddar cheese shredded
- pinch of Italian seasoning
- 1 tbsp. pizza sauce
- 1/2 avocado sliced
- 2 eggs boiled
- 1 tomato, halves
- 4 oz. fresh spinach leaves

Directions:

1. Warmth your Chaffle maker and grease with Cooking spray.
2. Whisk an egg in a bowl and beat with Italian seasoning and pizza sauce.
3. Add shredded cheese to the egg and spices mixture.
4. Pour 1 tbsp. shredded cheese in a Chaffle maker and Cooking for 30 sec.
5. Pour Chaffles batter in the Chaffle maker and close the lid.

6. Cooking chaffles for about 4 minutes until crispy and brown.
7. Carefully remove chaffles from the maker.
8. Serve on the bed of spinach with boil egg, avocado slice, and tomatoes.
9. Enjoy!

Nutrition:

Calories: 549

Total Fat: 49g

Carbs: 16g

Net Carbs: 11g

Fiber: 5g

Protein: 16g

Crispy Chaffles with Sausage

Preparation Time: 15 minutes

Cooking Time: 10 minutes

Servings: 2

Ingredients

- 1/2 cup cheddar cheese
- 1/2 tsp. baking powder
- 1/4 cup egg whites
- 2 tsp. pumpkin spice
- 1 egg, whole
- 2 chicken sausage
- 2 slice bacon
- salt and pepper to taste
- 1 tsp. avocado oil
1. Directions
2. Mix together all ingredients in a bowl.
3. Allow batter to sit while Chaffle iron warms.
4. Spray Chaffle iron with nonstick spray.
5. Pour batter in the Chaffle maker and Cooking according to the directions of the manufacturer.
6. Meanwhile, heat oil in a pan and fry the egg, according to your choice and transfer it to a plate.
7. In the same pan, fry bacon slice and sausage on medium heat for about 2-3 minutes until Cooked.

8. Once chaffles are cooked thoroughly, remove them from the maker.
9. Serve with fried egg, bacon slice, sausages and enjoy!

Nutrition:

Calories: 204

Total Fat: 11g

Total Carbs: 4.2g

Protein: 1.5g

Mini Breakfast Chaffles

Preparation Time: 30 minutes

Cooking Time: 15 minutes

Servings: 3

Ingredients:

- 6 tsp. coconut flour
- 1 tsp. stevia
- 1/4 tsp. baking powder
- 2 eggs
- 3 oz. cream cheese
- 1/2. tsp. vanilla extract
- 1 egg
- 6 slice bacon
- 2 oz. Raspberries for topping
- 2 oz. Blueberries for topping
- 2 oz. Strawberries for topping

Directions:

1. Heat up your square Chaffle maker and grease with cooking spray.
2. Mix together coconut flour, stevia, egg, baking powder, cheese and vanilla in mixing bowl.
3. Pour 1/2 of chaffles mixture in a Chaffle maker.
4. Close the lid and cooking the chaffles for about 3-5 minutes.

5. Meanwhile, fry bacon slices in pan on medium heat for about 2-3 minutes until Cooked and transfer them to plate.
6. In the same pan, fry eggs one by one in the leftover grease of bacon.
7. Once chaffles are cooked, carefully transfer them to plate.
8. Serve with fried eggs and bacon slice and berries on top.
9. Enjoy!

Nutrition:

Calories: 665

Net Carbs: 6.2g

Fat: 54g

Protein: 32g

Crispy Chaffles with Egg and Asparagus

Preparation Time: 15 minutes

Cooking Time: 10 minutes

Servings: 1

Ingredients:

- 1 egg
- 1/4 cup cheddar cheese
- 2 tbsps. almond flour
- 1/2 tsp. baking powder
- 1 egg
- 4-5 stalks asparagus
- 1 tsp. avocado oil

Directions:

1. Preheat Chaffle maker to medium-high heat.
2. Whisk together egg, Mozzarella cheese, almond flour, and baking powder
3. Pour chaffles mixture into the center of the Chaffle iron. Close the Chaffle maker and let cooking for 3-5 minutes or until Chaffle is golden brown and set.
4. Remove chaffles from the Chaffle maker and serve.
5. Meanwhile, heat oil in a nonstick pan.

6. Once the pan is hot, fry asparagus for about 4-5 minutes until golden brown.
7. Poach the egg in boil water for about 2-3 minutes.
8. Once chaffles are cooked, remove from the maker.
9. Serve chaffles with the poached egg and asparagus.

Nutrition:

Calories: 287

Total Fat: 19g

Total Carbs: 6.5g

Protein: 6.8g

Coconut Chaffles

Preparation Time: 10 minutes

Cooking Time: 5 minutes

Servings: 2

Ingredients:

- 1 egg
- 1 oz. cream cheese,
- 1 oz. cheddar cheese
- 2 tbsps. coconut flour
- 1 tsp. stevia
- 1 tbsp. coconut oil, melted
- 1/2 tsp. coconut extract
- 2 eggs, soft boil for serving

Directions:

1. Heat your Chaffle maker and grease with cooking spray.
2. Mix together all chaffles ingredients in a bowl.
3. Pour chaffle batter in a preheated Chaffle maker.
4. Close the lid.
5. Cooking chaffles for about 2-3 minutes until golden brown.
6. Serve with boil egg and enjoy

Nutrition:

Calories: 331

Protein: 11.84 g

Fat: 30.92 g

Carbohydrates: 1.06g

Keto Basil Buns

Preparation Time: 10 minutes

Cooking Time: 20 minutes

Servings: 8

Ingredients

- 4 eggs
- 3/4 cup almond flour
- 6 Tbsp. butter
- 6 garlic cloves, crushed
- 5 1/2 oz. parmesan cheese, grated
- 3/4 cup of water
- 1 cup fresh basil, chopped
- Salt to taste

Directions

1. Heat water until boiling and add the butter and salt.
2. Add flour and mix until smooth. Then remove from heat.
3. Crack eggs into the dough one at a time, mixing after each egg.
4. Add garlic, basil, and Parmesan. Mix until smooth.
5. Set a baking sheet with parchment paper and place the dough on it one spoonful at a time to form buns.
6. Bake at 392F for 20 minutes.
7. Serve.

Nutrition:

Calories: 186

Fat: 15g

Carb: 1.4g

Protein: 9.6g

English Muffin

Preparation Time: 10 minutes

Cooking Time: 5 minutes

Servings: 2

Ingredients

- 1/4 cup almond flour
- 1 Tbsp. coconut flour
- 1/8 tsp. baking soda
- 1/8 tsp. salt
- 1 egg white
- 1/2 tsp. oil
- 2 Tbsp. warm water
- Butter, jam, or scrambled egg for serving

Directions

1. Add the flours, baking soda, and salt in a small ramekin and mix well with a fork.
2. Add the egg white, oil, and water, mix well.
3. Flatten the batter, so it is even on top.
4. For 2 minutes, microwave the ramekin.
5. To slide out the muffin, turn the ramekin upside down.
6. Slice it into 2 muffin halves and toast each slice.
7. Spread with butter or sugar-free jam or scrambled egg.

8. Serve.

Nutrition:

Calories: 114

Fat: 1g

Carb: 5g

Protein: 5g

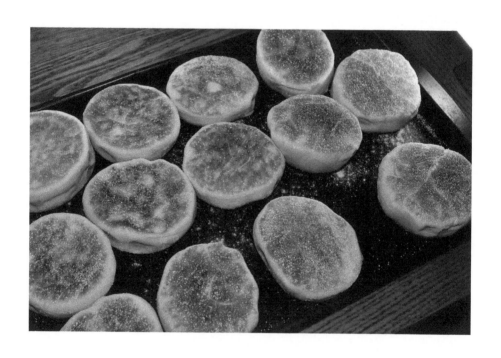

Egg-free Coconut Flour Chaffles

Preparation Time: 5 minutes

Cooking Time: 10 minutes

Servings: 2

Ingredients:

- 1 tablespoon flaxseed meal
- 21/2 tablespoons water
- 1/4 cup Mozzarella cheese, shredded
- 1 tablespoon cream cheese, softened
- 2 tablespoons coconut flour

Directions:

1. Preheat a Chaffle iron and then grease it.
2. In a bowl, place the flaxseed meal and water and mix well.
3. Set aside for about 5 minutes or until thickened.
4. In the bowl of flaxseed mixture, add the remaining Ingredients: and mix until well merged.
5. Set half of the mixture into preheated Chaffle iron and Cooking for about 3-minutes or until golden brown.
6. Repeat with the remaining mixture. Serve warm.

Nutrition:

Calories: 76

Net Carb: 2.3g

Fat: 4.2g

Saturated Fat: 2.1g

Carbohydrates: 6.3g

Dietary Fiber: 4g

Sugar: 0.1g

Protein: 3g

Simple Chaffle Toast

Preparation Time: 5 minutes

Cooking Time: 5 minutes

Servings: 2

Ingredients:

- 1 large egg
- 1/2 cup shredded cheddar cheese

For Topping

- 1 egg
- 3-4 spinach leaves
- 1/4 cup boil and shredded chicken

Directions:

1. Preheat your square Chaffle maker on medium-high heat.
2. Mix together egg and cheese in a bowl and make two chaffles in a chaffle maker.
3. Once chaffle are Cooked, carefully remove them from the maker.
4. Serve with spinach, boiled chicken, and fried egg.
5. Serve hot and enjoy!

Nutrition:

Protein: 99

Fat: 153

Carbohydrates: 3

Protein: 5.7g

Sausage Chaffles

Preparation Time: 5 minutes

Cooking Time: 1 hour

Servings: 12

Ingredients:

- 1 pound gluten-free bulk Italian sausage crumbled
- 1 organic egg, beaten
- 1 cup sharp Cheddar cheese, shredded
- 1/4 cup Parmesan cheese, grated
- 1 cup almond flour
- 2 teaspoons organic baking powder

Directions:

1. Preheat a mini Chaffle iron and then grease It.
2. In a medium bowl, set all Ingredients: and with your hands, mix until well combined.
3. Place about 3 tablespoons of the mixture 1 into preheated Chaffle iron and Cooking for about 3 minutes or until golden brown.
4. Carefully, flip the chaffle and Cooking for about 2 minutes or until golden brown.
5. Repeat with the remaining mixture.
6. Serve warm.

Nutrition:

Calories: 238

Net Carb: 1 .2 g

Fat: 1 9.6 g

Saturated Fat: 6.1g

Carbohydrates: 2.2g

Sugar 0.4g

Protein 10.8g

Egg and Chives Chaffle Sandwich Roll

Preparation Time: 5 minutes

Cooking Time: 10 minutes

Servings: 2

Ingredients:

- 2 tablespoons mayonnaise
- 1 hard-boiled egg, chopped
- 1 tablespoon chives, chopped
- 2 basic chaffles

Directions:

1. In a bowl, mix the mayo, egg and chives.
2. Spread the mixture on top of the chaffles.
3. Roll the chaffle.

Nutrition:

Calories 258

Total Fat 12g

Saturated Fat 2.8g

Cholesterol 171mg

Sodium 271mg

Potassium 71mg

Total Carbohydrate 7

Protein 5.9g

Total Sugars 2.3g

Savory Chaffles Bacon and Jalapeno Chaffles

Preparation Time: 5 minutes

Cooking Time: 15 minutes

Servings: 5

Ingredients:

- 3 tablespoons coconut flour
- 1 teaspoon organic baking powder
- 1/4 teaspoon salt
- 1/2 cup cream cheese, softened
- 3 large organic eggs
- 1 cup sharp Cheddar cheese, shredded
- 1 jalapeno pepper, seeded and chopped
- 3 Cooked bacon slices, crumbled

Directions:

1. Preheat a mini Chaffle iron and then grease it.
2. In a small bowl, merge the flour, baking powder and salt and mix well.
3. In a large bowl, place the cream cheese and beat until light and fluffy.
4. Add the eggs and Cheddar cheese and beat until well combined.
5. Add the flour mixture and beat until combined.

6. Fold in the jalapeno pepper.

7. Divide the mixture into 5 portions.

8. Place 1 portion of the mixture into preheated Chaffle iron and Cooking for about 5 minutes or until golden brown.

9. Repeat with the remaining mixture.

10.Serve warm with the topping of bacon pieces.

Nutrition:

Calories: 249

Net Carb: 2.99

Fat: 20.3g

Saturated Fat: 5g

Carbohydrates: 4.8g

Sugar: 0.5g

Protein: 12.7g

Lightning Source UK Ltd.
Milton Keynes UK
UKHW020644100621
385263UK00001B/176